Place a special photo here.

hello, baby

a keepsake book

Parragon.

Dedication

....

....

....

....

Published 2024 by Parragon Books, Ltd.

Copyright © 2024 Cottage Door Press, LLC
5005 Newport Drive, Rolling Meadows, Illinois 60008

Illustrated by Rose Halsey

All rights reserved. No part of this publication may be reproduced, stored in a retrieval system, or transmitted, in any form or by any means, electronic, mechanical, photocopying, recording, or otherwise, without the prior permission of the copyright holder.

ISBN 978-1-64638-914-8

Parragon Books is an imprint of Cottage Door Press, LLC. Parragon® and the Parragon® logo are registered trademarks of Cottage Door Press, LLC.

Contents

A Letter to You Before You Are Born	4
Our Family Tree	6
About Our Family	7
The Day You Were Born	8
Welcome Home	10
Ten Tiny Fingers and Ten Tiny Toes	11
Your Name	12
First Things First	14
Milestones	16
One Month	18
Two Months	20
Three Months	22
Four Months	24
Five Months	26
Six Months	28
Seven Months	30
Eight Months	32
Nine Months	34
Ten Months	36
Eleven Months	38
Twelve Months	40
Happy First Birthday!	42
A Year of You	44
Wishes for You	45
You're Two Cool!	46
Two Terrific Years	48
Young, Wild, and Three!	50
Three Years Strong	52
Favorite Places	54
Beginning with Books	56
Animal Friends	58
Holiday Moments	60
A Letter to Future You	62

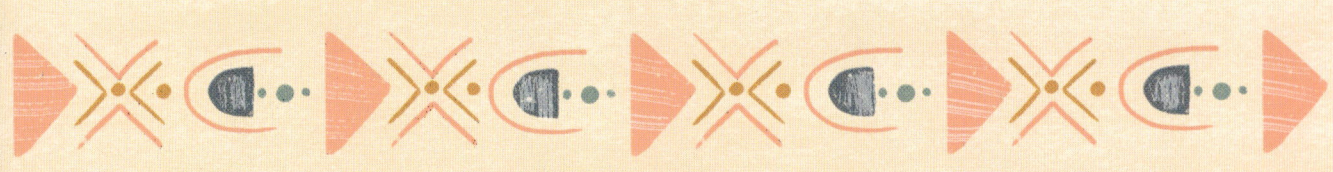

A Letter to You Before You Are Born

These are our hopes, dreams, wishes, and predictions about future you.

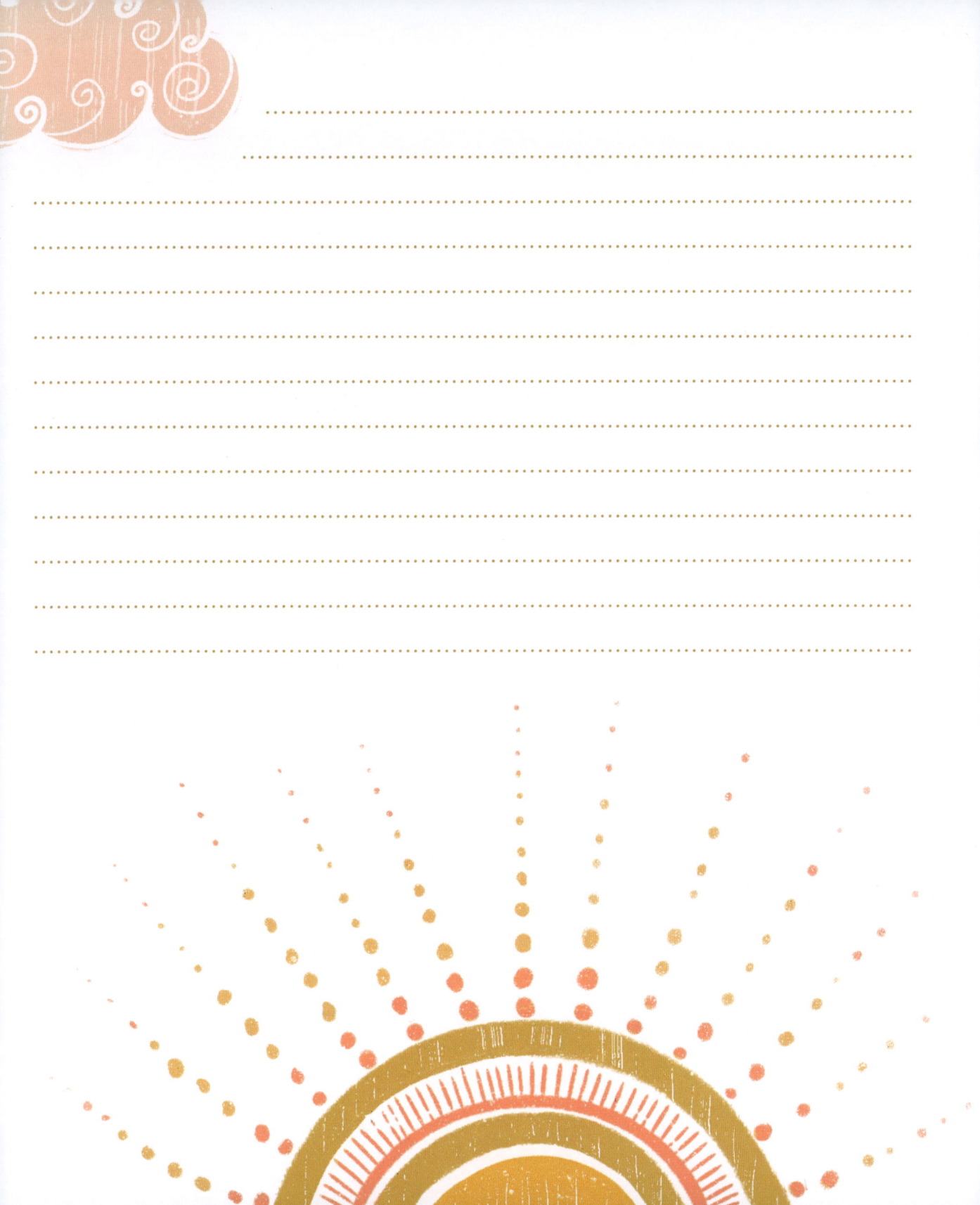

Our Family Tree

Use stickers to add names to the tree.

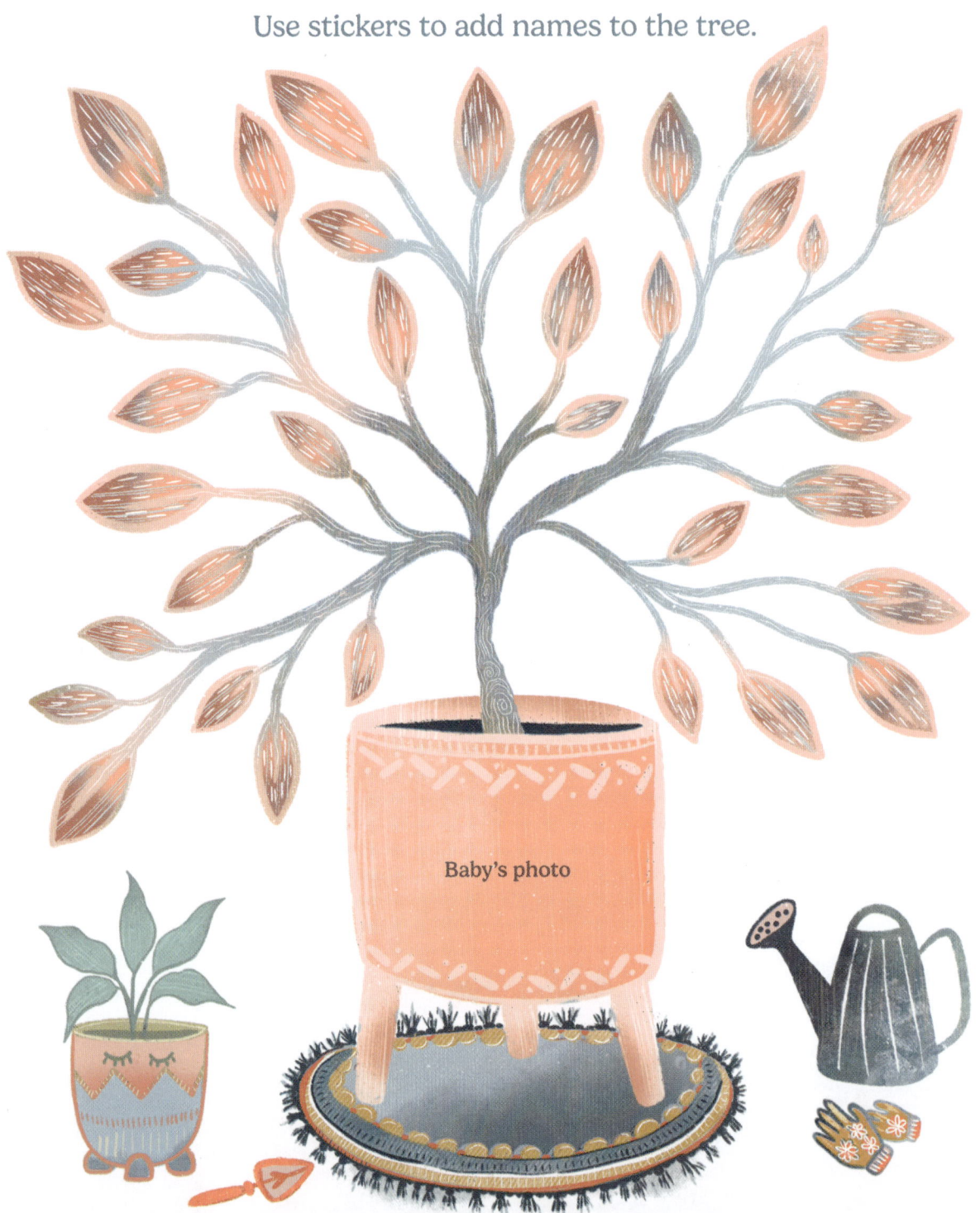

About Our Family

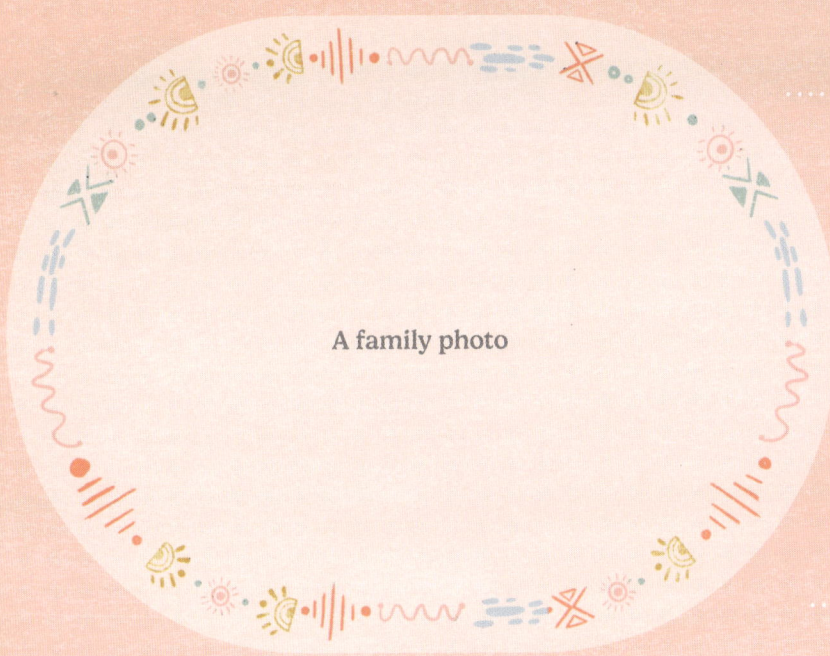

A family photo

More special people we want you to know about:

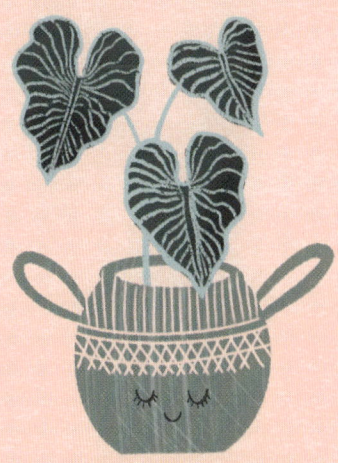

The Day You Were Born

Your Birth Story

Baby's first photo

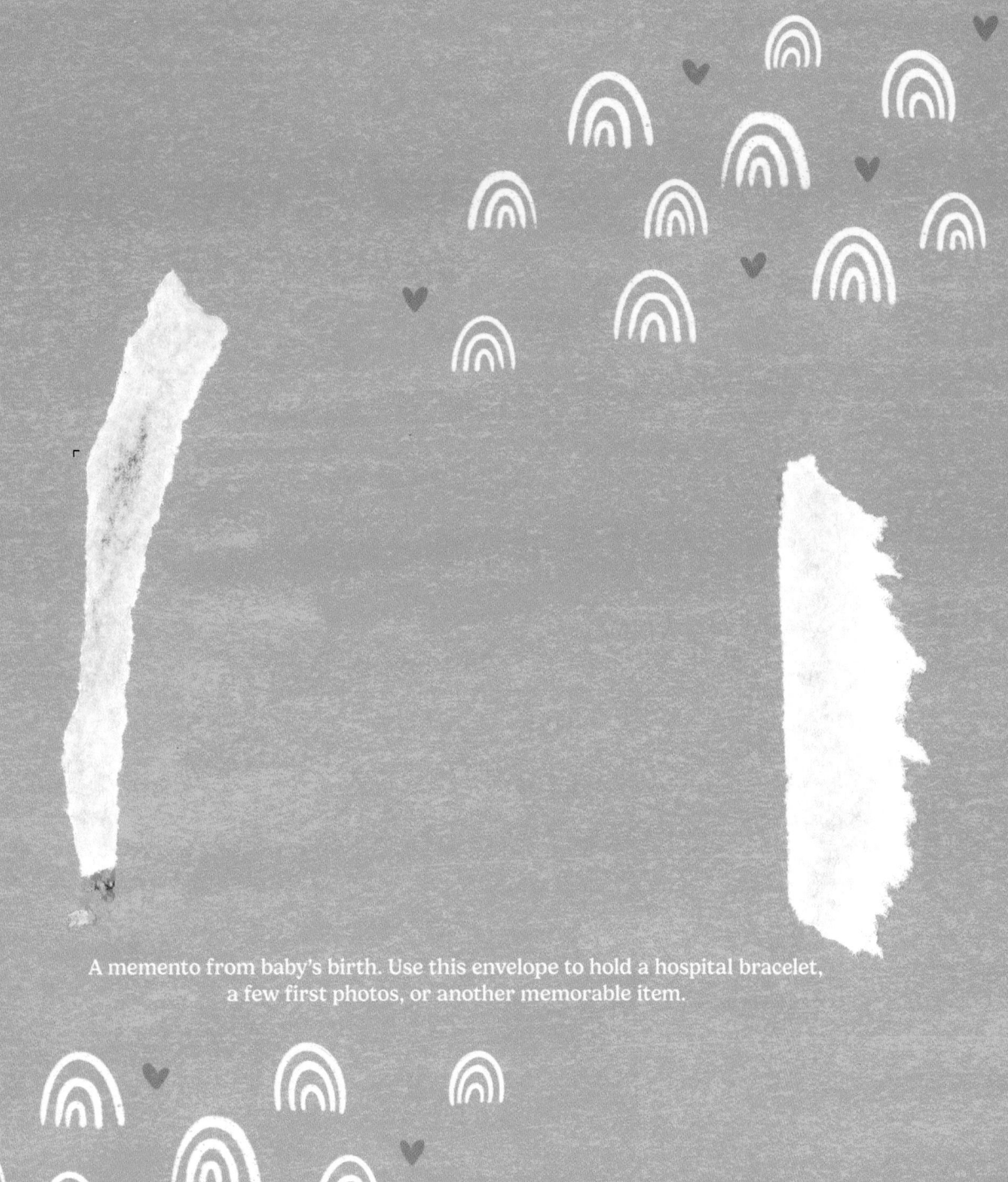

A memento from baby's birth. Use this envelope to hold a hospital bracelet, a few first photos, or another memorable item.

Welcome Home

You came home ....
....
....
....
....
....

A photo of baby at home

A photo of baby meeting people at home

....
....
....
....

Ten Tiny Fingers and Ten Tiny Toes

Place baby's handprint and footprint on this page.

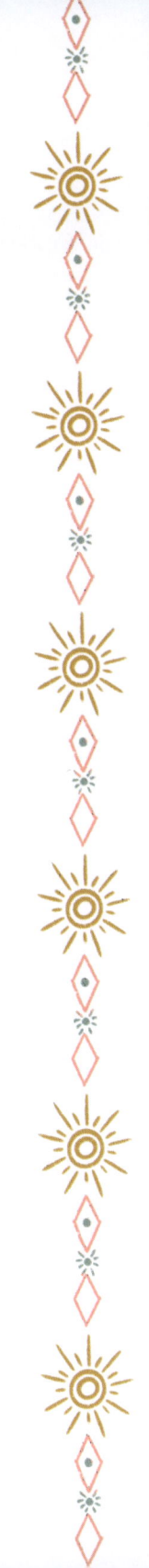

Your Name

Your full name is ....

Your name means ....
....
....
....

The inspiration for your name was ....
....
....
....

You share your name with ....
....
....

Other names we considered were ....
....
....

Our first photo
as a new family

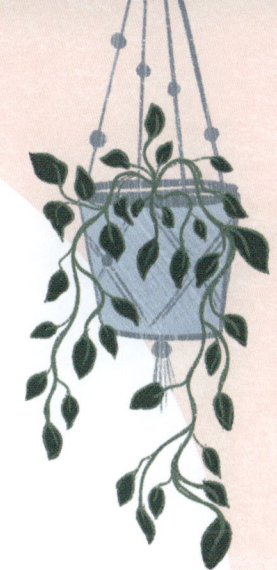

A photo of baby with
someone special

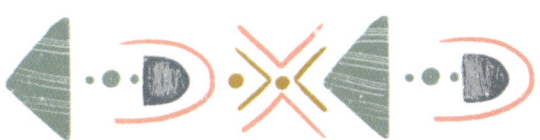

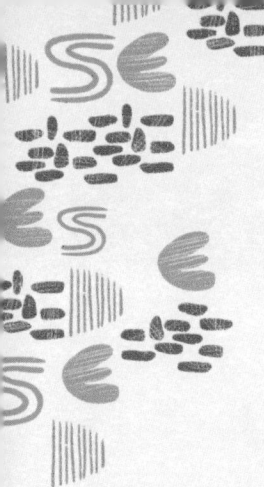
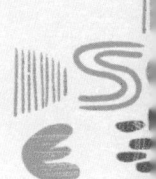

First Things First

These are some of your most memorable "firsts."

A photo of a special "first"
(baby's first bath, meeting someone
for the first time, or a first smile)

....

....

....

....

....

Your first solid food

....
....
....
....
....
....

A photo of baby walking

A photo of baby eating something yummy

Your first steps

....
....
....
....
....
....
....

Milestones

You first smiled

You first laughed

Your first bath

Your first doctor's appointment

Your first outing

You first sat up

You first rolled over

You first slept through the night

You first waved

You first crawled

Your first bottle

You first met a special family member

One Month

On ....

you turned one month old!

A photo at one month old!

You weigh ....

and are .... inches tall.

You love
....
....

You can
....
....
....

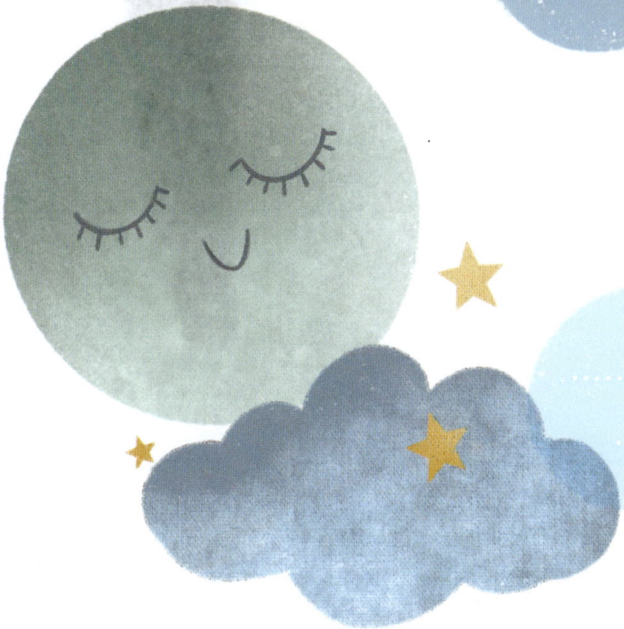

You don't like
....
....
....

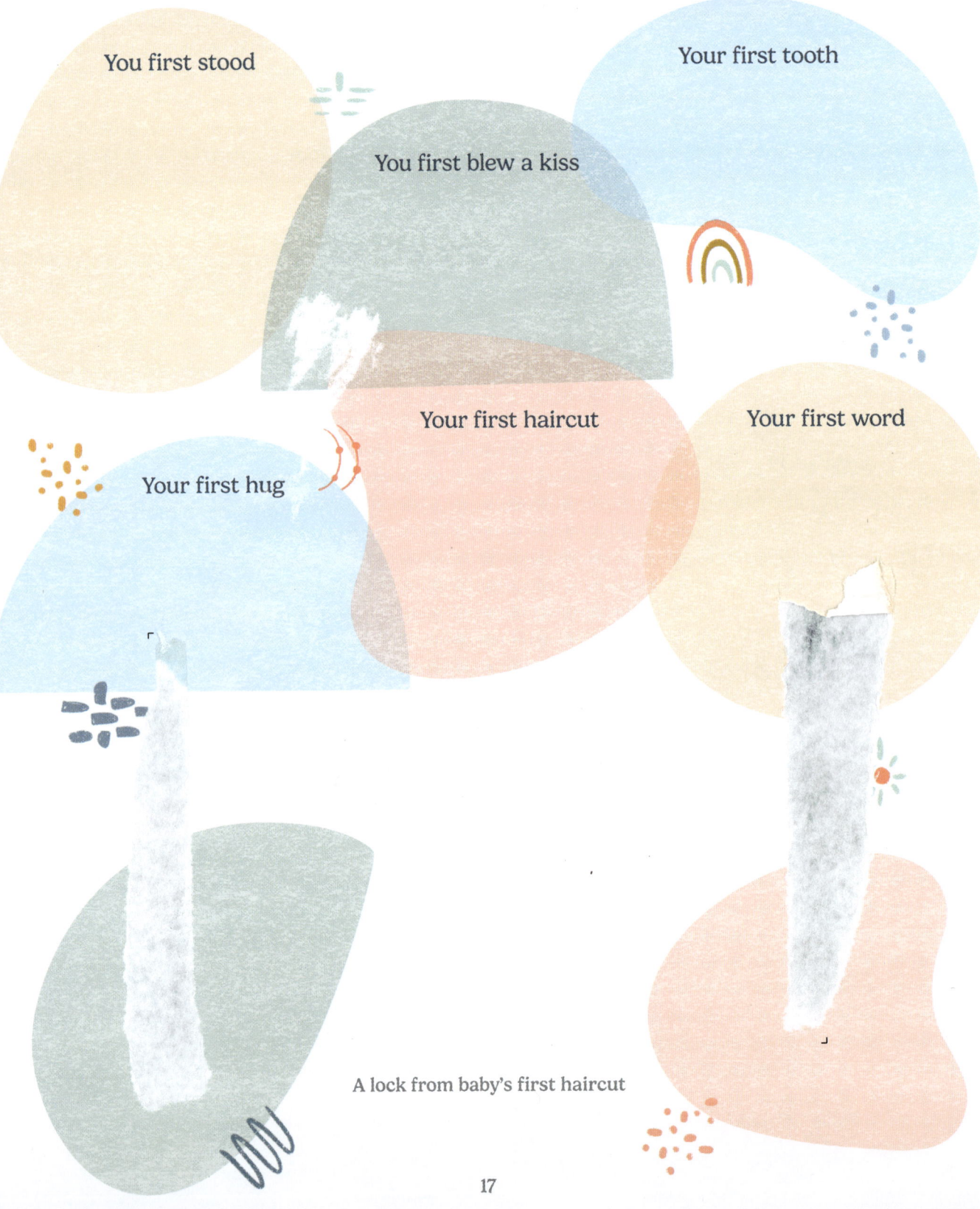

Favorite book: ....

....

Favorite toy: ....

....

Favorite activity: ....

....

Favorite song: ....

....

A photo of a favorite one-month memory

Our family's favorite moments with you this month: ....

....

....

....

Two Months

On ....
you turned two months old!

You weigh ....
and are .... inches tall.

A photo at two months old!

You love
....
....
....
....
....
....

You can
....
....
....
....

You don't like ....
....
....
....
....

Favorite book: ………………………… Favorite activity: …………………………
………………………………………………… …………………………………………………
Favorite toy: ………………………… Favorite song: …………………………
………………………………………………… …………………………………………………

A photo of a favorite two-month memory

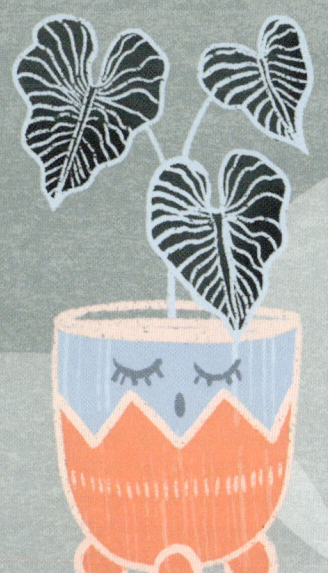

Our family's favorite moments with you this month:
……………………………………………………………………………………………
……………………………………………………………………………………………
……………………………………………………………………………………………
……………………………………………………………………………………………

Three Months

On ....
you turned three months old!

You weigh ....
and are .... inches tall.

A photo at three months old!

You love ....
....
....

You don't like ....
....
....
....
....

You can ....
....
....
....
....

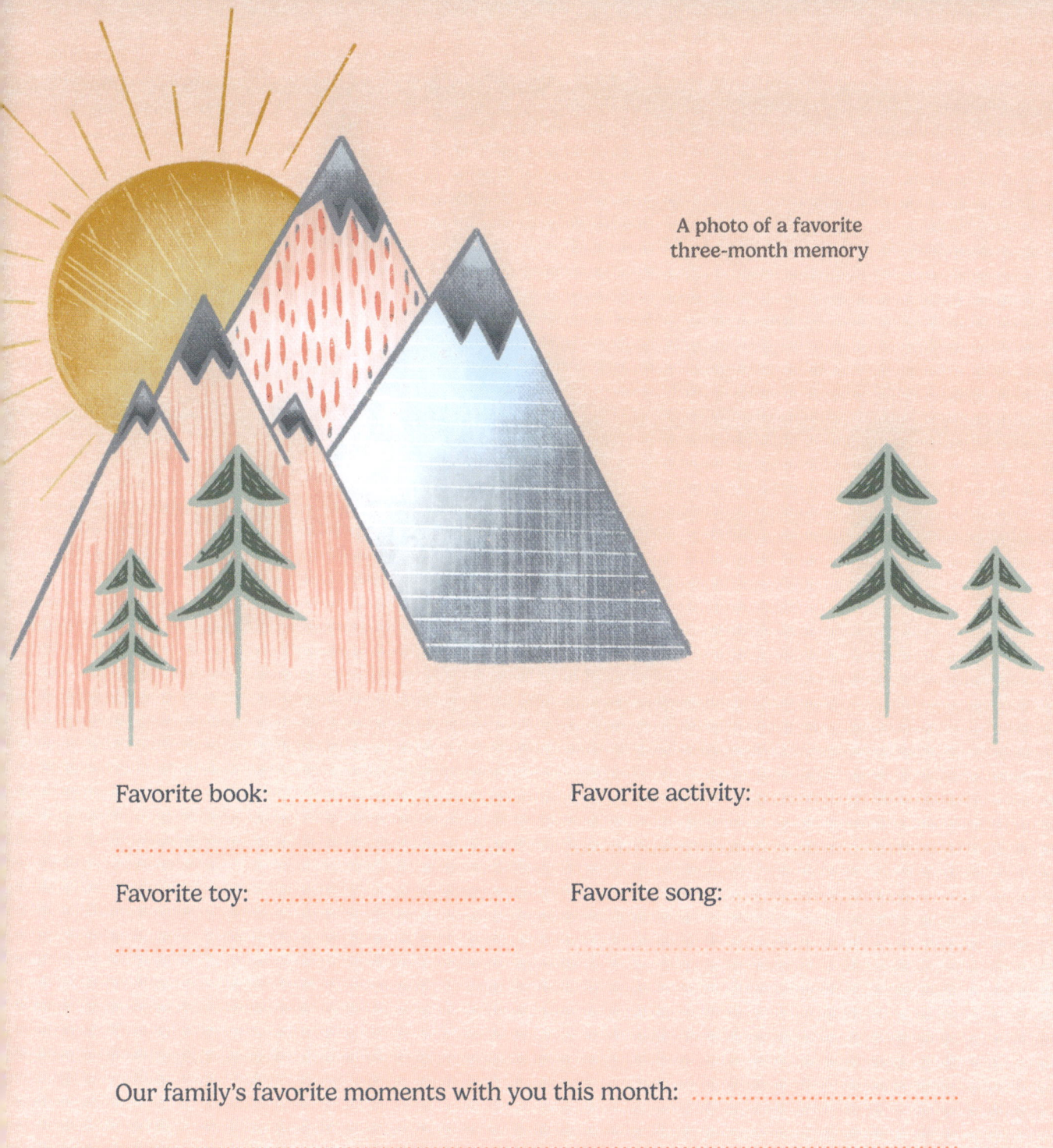

A photo of a favorite three-month memory

Favorite book: ....

Favorite toy: ....

Favorite activity: ....

Favorite song: ....

Our family's favorite moments with you this month: ....

Four Months

On ....
you turned four months old!

You weigh ....
and are .... inches tall.

You love ....
....
....
....

You don't like ....
....
....
....
....

You can ....
....
....
....
....
....
....

A photo at four months old!

Favorite book: ....

....

Favorite toy: ....

....

Favorite activity: ....

....

Favorite song: ....

....

Our family's favorite moments with you this month: ....

....

....

....

....

A photo of a favorite four-month memory

Five Months

On ....
you turned five months old!

You weigh ....
and are .... inches tall.

A photo at five months old!

You love

....
....
....
....

You don't like

....
....
....
....

You can

....
....
....
....

Favorite book: ....
....

Favorite toy: ....
....

Favorite activity: ....
....

Favorite song: ....
....

Our family's favorite moments with you this month: ....
....
....
....
....
....

A photo of a favorite five-month memory

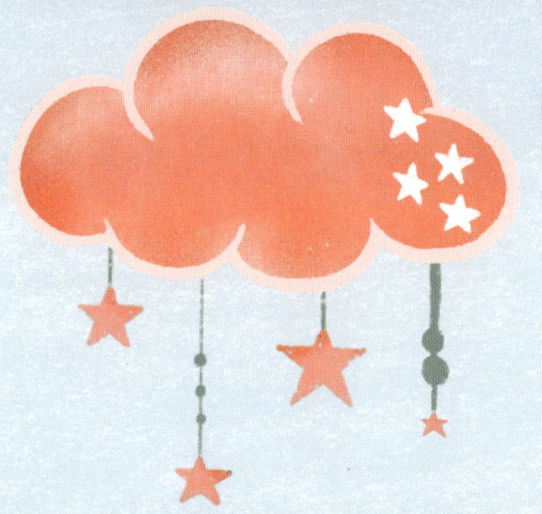

Six Months

On ....
you turned six months old!

You weigh ....
and are .... inches tall.

You love ....
....
....
....

A photo at six months old!

You can ....
....
....
....
....

You don't like ....
....
....
....
....

Favorite book: ....　　Favorite activity: ....

....　　..

Favorite toy: ....　　Favorite song: ....

....　　..

A photo of a favorite six-month memory

Our family's favorite moments with you this month: ....
....
....
....
....
....
....
....

Seven Months

On ....
you turned seven months old!

You weigh ....
and are .... inches tall.

A photo at seven months old!

You love ....
....
....
....

You don't like ....
....
....
....

You can ....
....
....
....

Favorite book: ....   Favorite activity: ....
....
Favorite food: ....   Favorite song: ....
....

A photo of a favorite
seven-month memory

Our family's favorite moments with you this month: ....
....
....

Eight Months

On .... you turned eight months old!

You weigh ....
and are .... inches tall.

You love ....
....
....
....

You don't like ....
....
....
....

You can ....
....
....
....
....
....
....

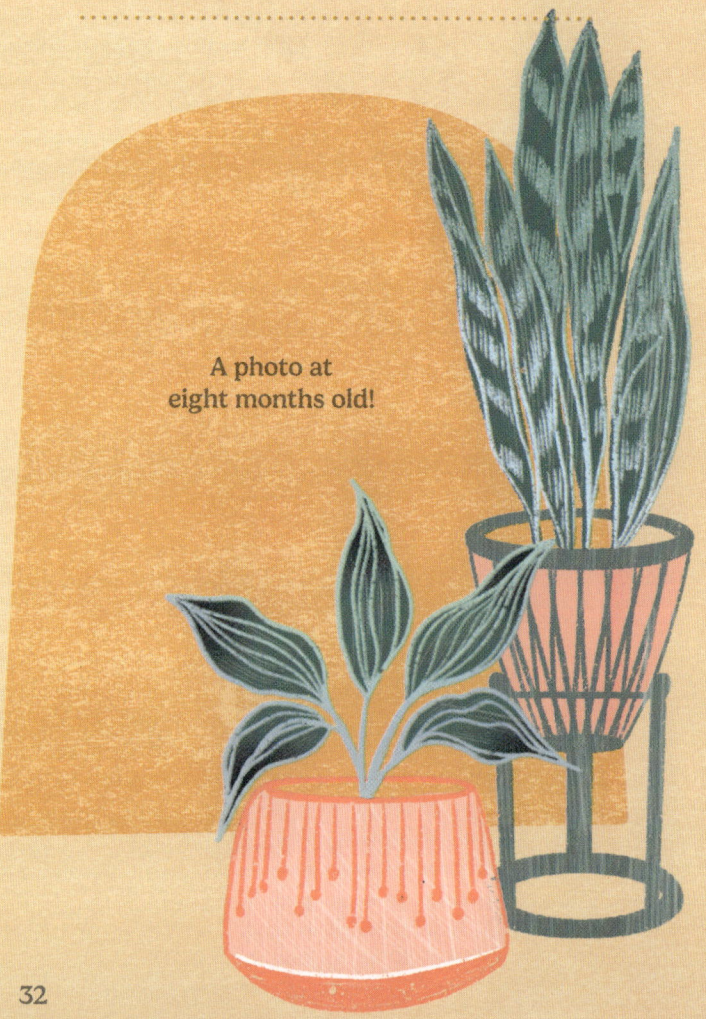

A photo at eight months old!

Favorite book: ....
....
Favorite food: ....
....
Favorite activity: ....
....
Favorite song: ....
....

Our family's favorite moments
with you this month: ....
....
....
....
....
....

A photo of a favorite eight-month memory

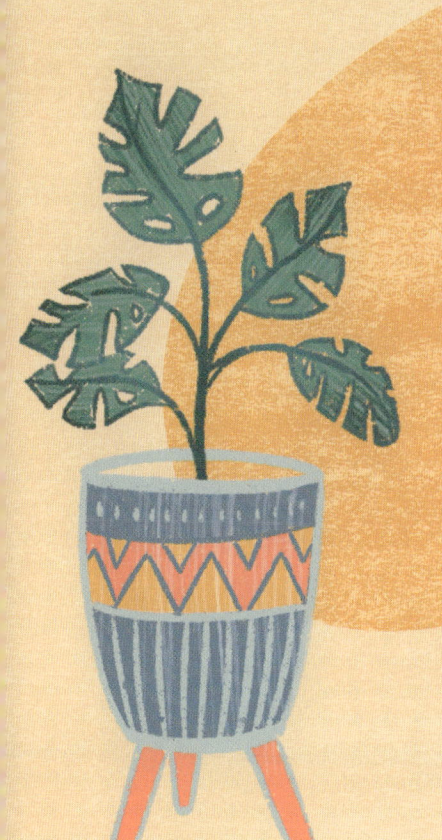
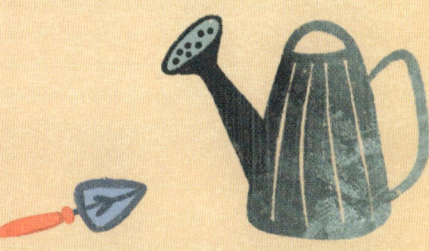

Nine Months

On ....
you turned nine months old!

You weigh ....
and are .... inches tall.

You love ....
....
....
....

A photo at nine months old!

You don't like ....
....
....
....

You can ....
....
....
....

Favorite book: ....

....

Favorite food: ....

....

Favorite activity: ....

....

Favorite song: ....

....

Our family's favorite moments with you this month: ....

....

....

....

....

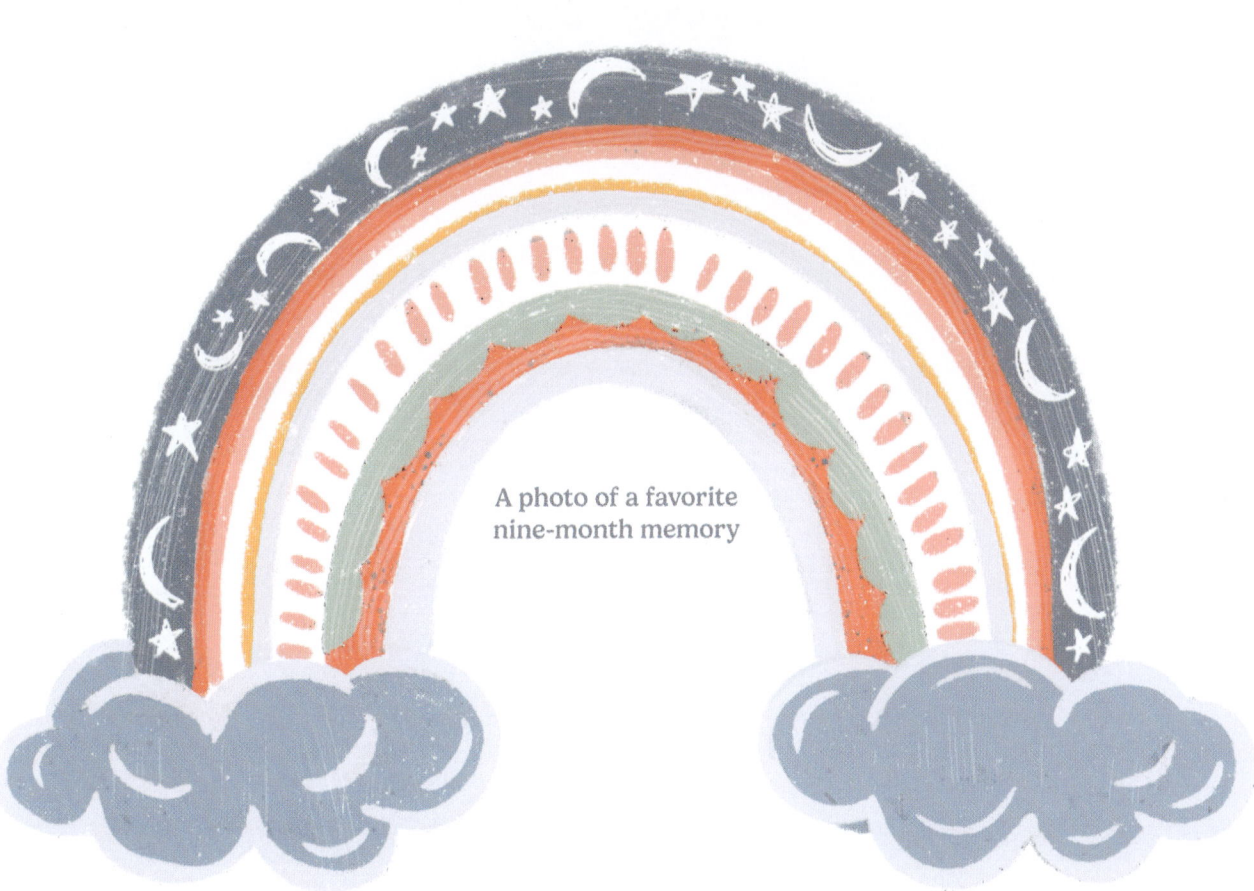

A photo of a favorite nine-month memory

Ten Months

On ....
you turned ten months old!

You weigh ....
and are .... inches tall.

A photo at ten months old!

You love
....
....
....
....

You can
....
....
....
....
....

You don't like
....
....
....
....

Favorite book: …………………………. Favorite activity: ……………………….

……………………………………………. ……………………………………………….

Favorite food: …………………………. Favorite song: ………………………….

…………………………………………….. ……………………………………………….

A photo of a favorite ten-month memory

Our family's favorite moments with you this month: ……………………………

………………………………………………………………………………………………………

………………………………………………………………………………………………………

Eleven Months

On ....
you turned eleven months old!

You weigh ....
and are .... inches tall.

A photo at eleven months old!

You love
....
....
....
....

You don't like ....
....
....
....
....

You can ....
....
....
....
....

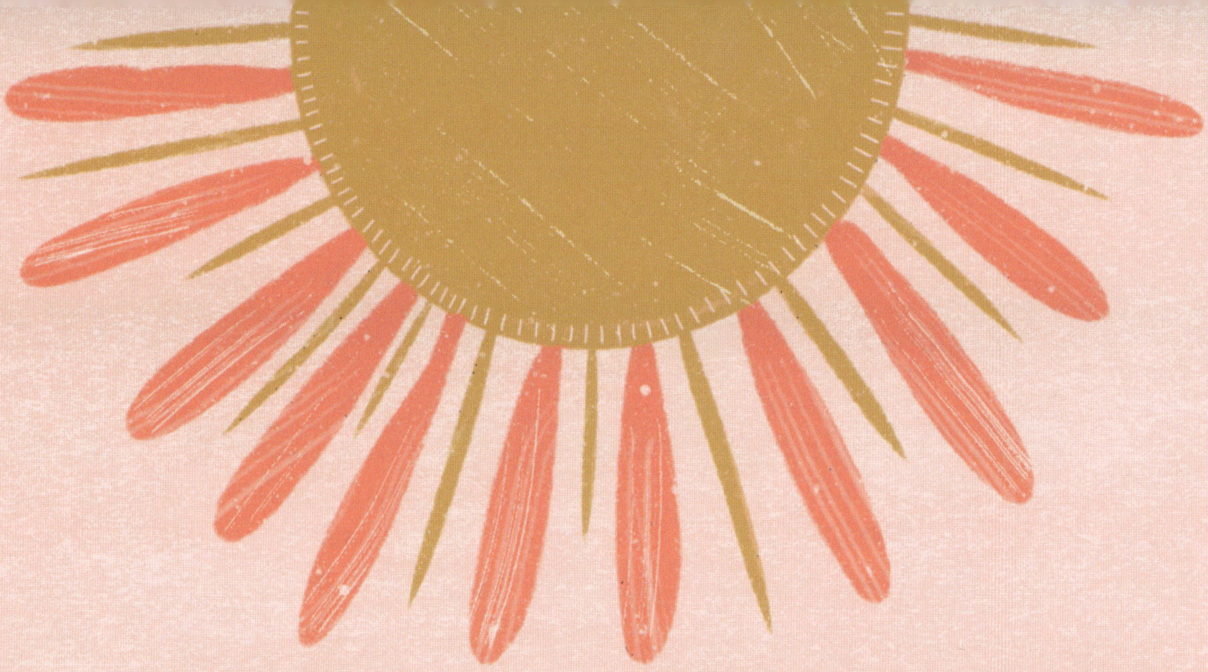

A photo of a favorite eleven-month memory

Favorite book: ....   Favorite activity: ....
....

Favorite food: ....   Favorite song: ....
....

Our family's favorite moments with you this month: ....
....
....

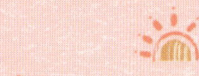

Twelve Months

On ....
you turned twelve months old!

You weigh ....
and are .... inches tall.

You like

....
....
....
....
....

You don't like

....
....
....
....
....

You can

....
....
....
....
....

A photo at twelve months old!

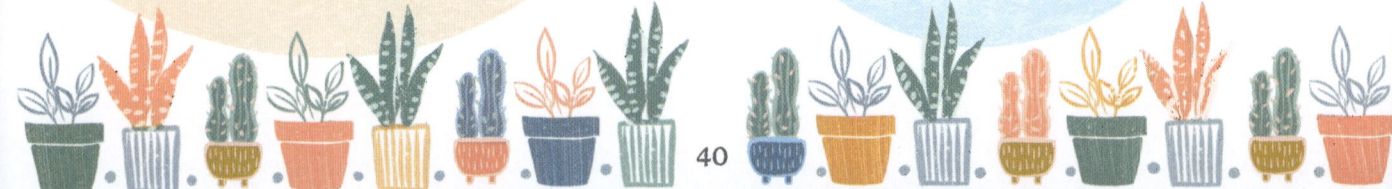

Favorite book: ....
....
Favorite food: ....
....

Our family's favorite moments with you this month:
....
....
....
....
....
....

Favorite activity: ....
....
....
Favorite song: ....
....
....

A photo of a favorite twelve-month memory

....
....

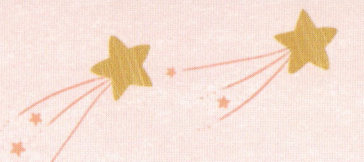 

Happy First Birthday!

A photo of a favorite birthday memory

This is how we celebrated your very first birthday: ....
....
....
....
....
....
....

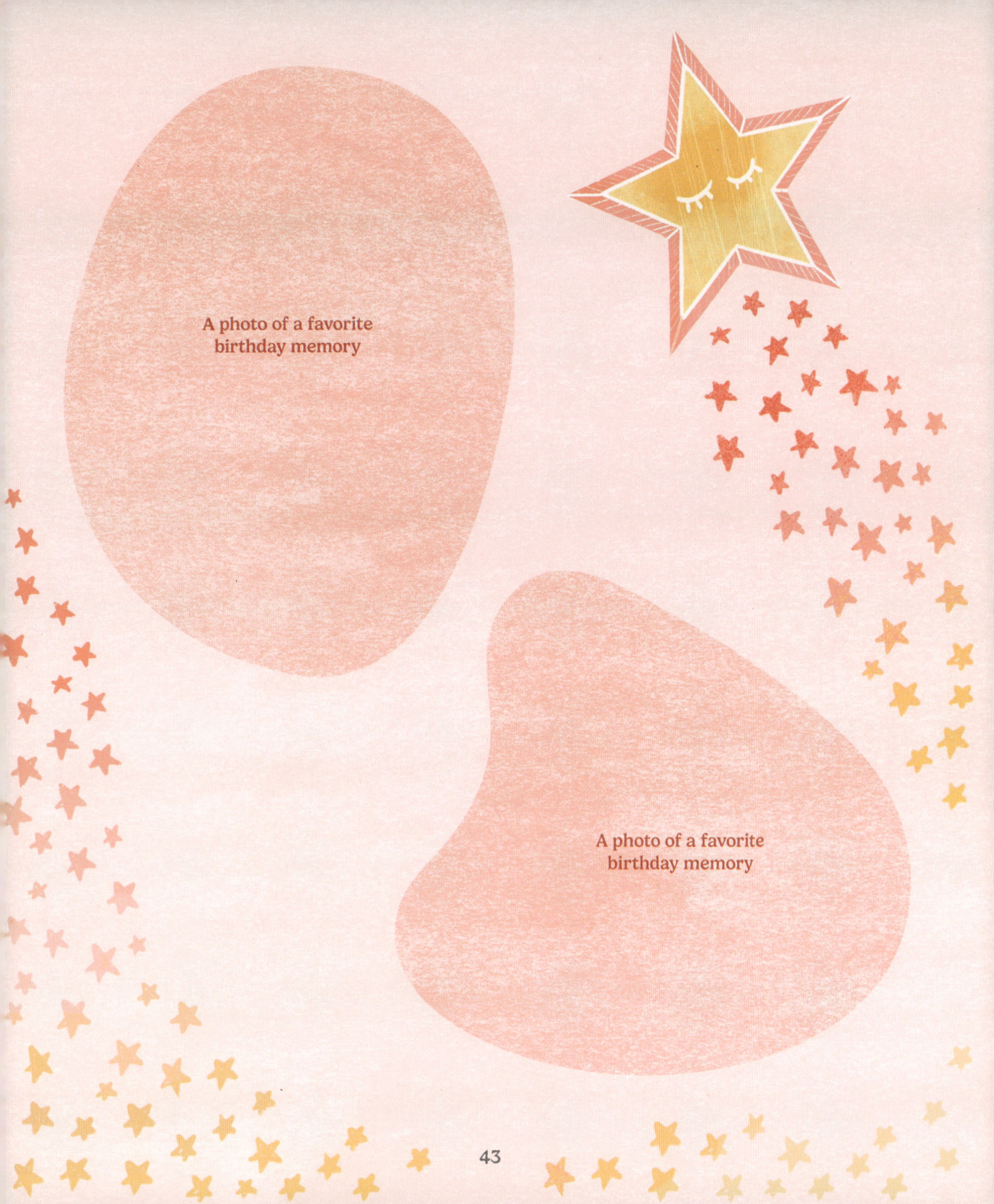

A Year of You

Here are some things we've learned after your first year.

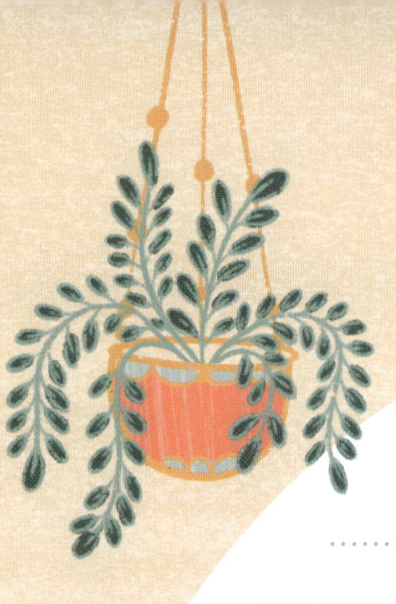

You taught us
....
....
....
....

You make others laugh by ....
....
....
....

Times when you tried really hard: ....
....
....
....

Ways you wondered about the world:
....
....
....
....

Moments when you were sweet: ....
....
....
....

Words you can say: ....
....
....

A favorite photo from baby's first year

Wishes for You

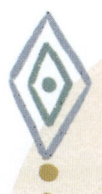

We hope you

We hope you can

We hope you get

We hope you learn

We hope you love

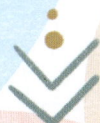

We hope you find

We hope you never forget

We hope you become

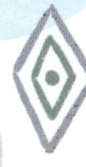

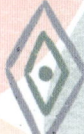

We hope you grow

We hope you inherit

You're Two Cool!

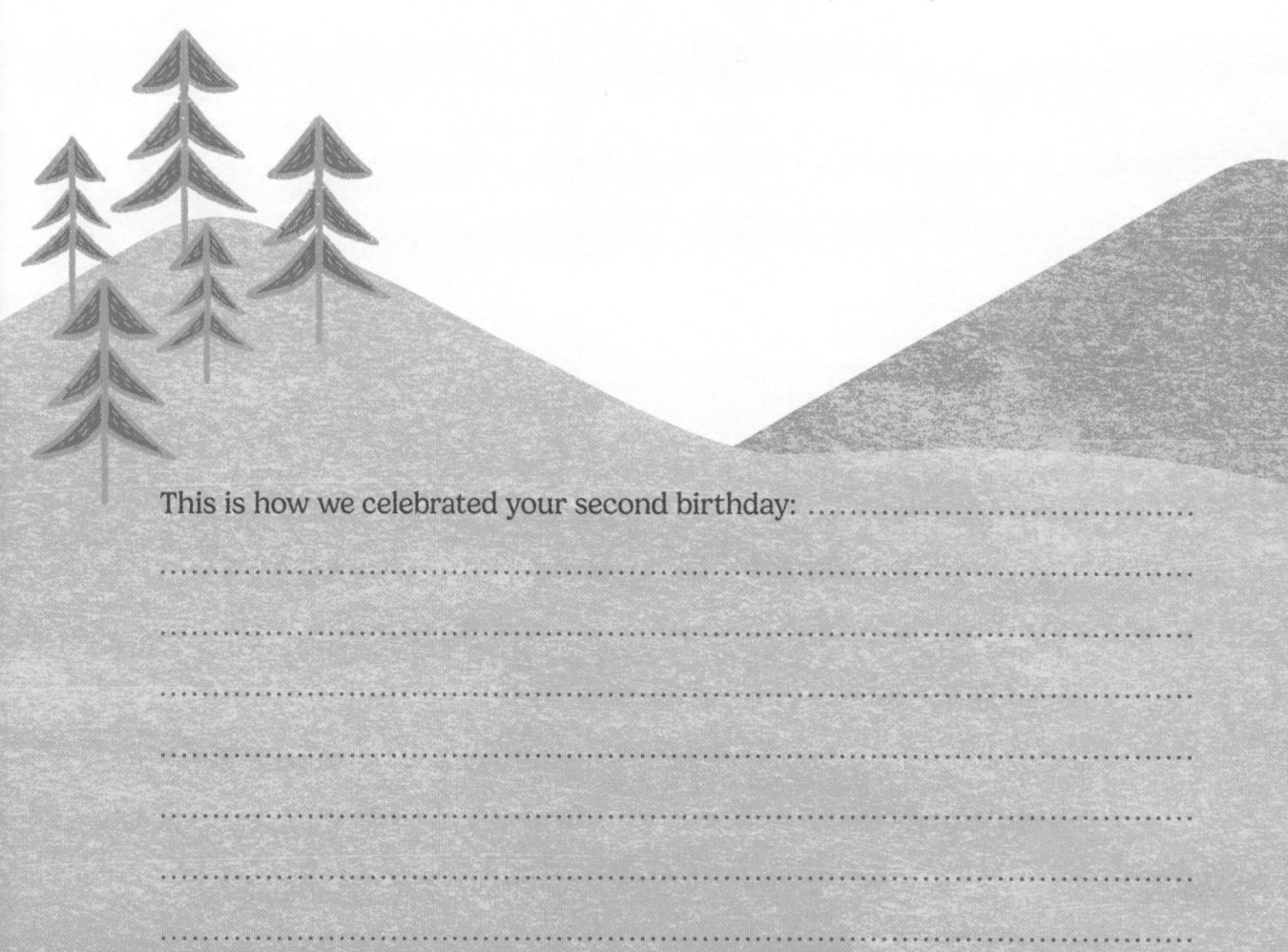

A photo of a favorite second birthday memory

This is how we celebrated your second birthday: ....
....
....
....
....
....
....

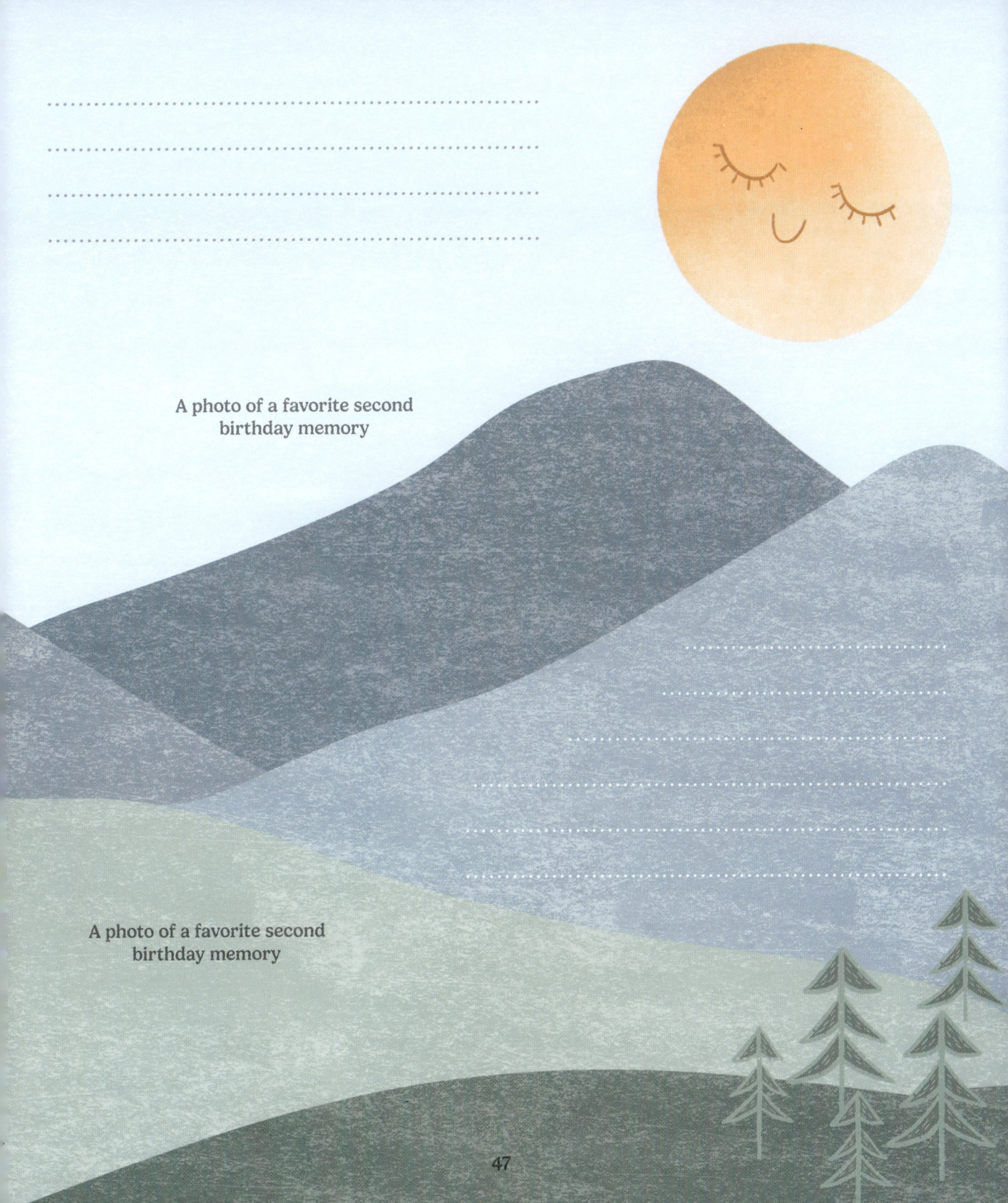

A photo of a favorite second birthday memory

A photo of a favorite second birthday memory

Two Terrific Years

These are some highlights from your second year.

You taught us ....
....
....
....

A favorite photo from baby's second year

You make others laugh by ....
....
....

Times when you tried really hard: ....
....
....
....

New friends you've made: ....
....
....
....

Ways you explored the world: ....
....
....
....

Funniest things you've said: ....
....
....

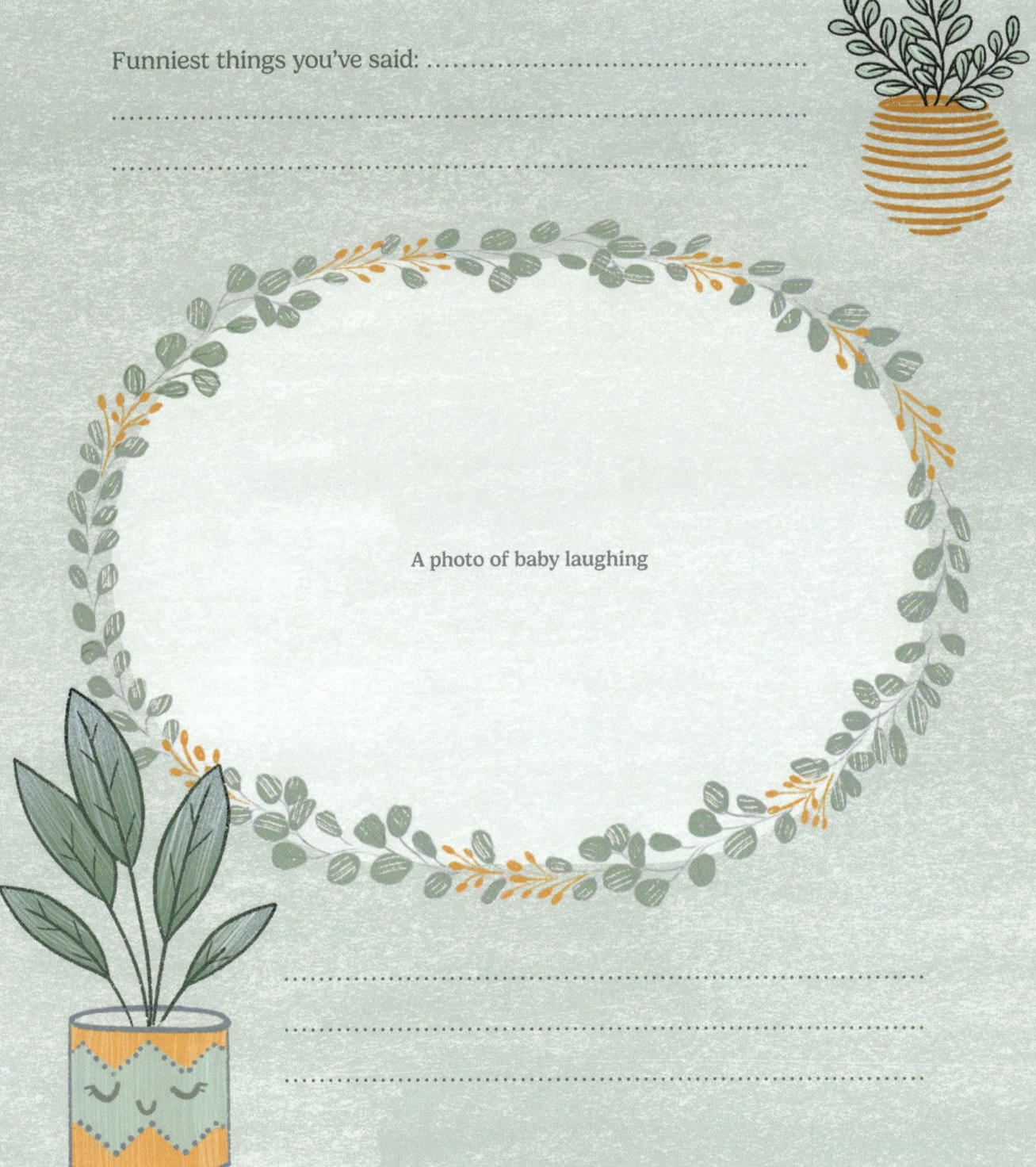

A photo of baby laughing

....
....
....

Young, Wild, and Three!

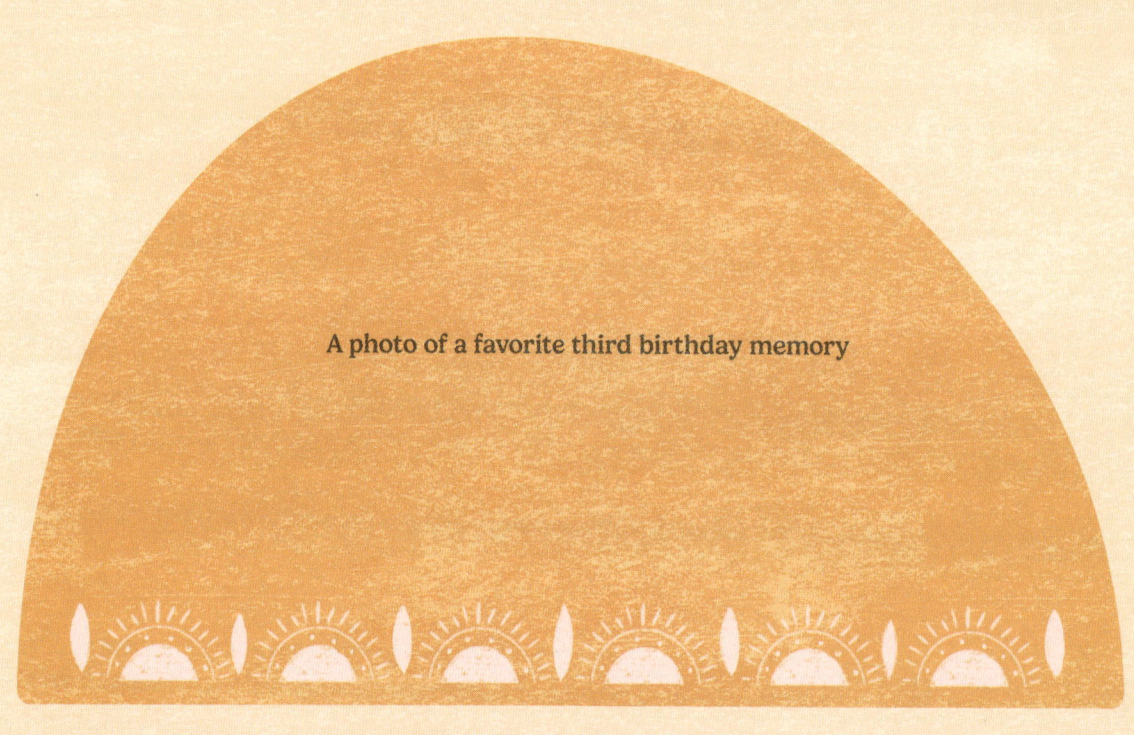

A photo of a favorite third birthday memory

This is how we celebrated your third birthday: ....
....
....
....
....
....
....

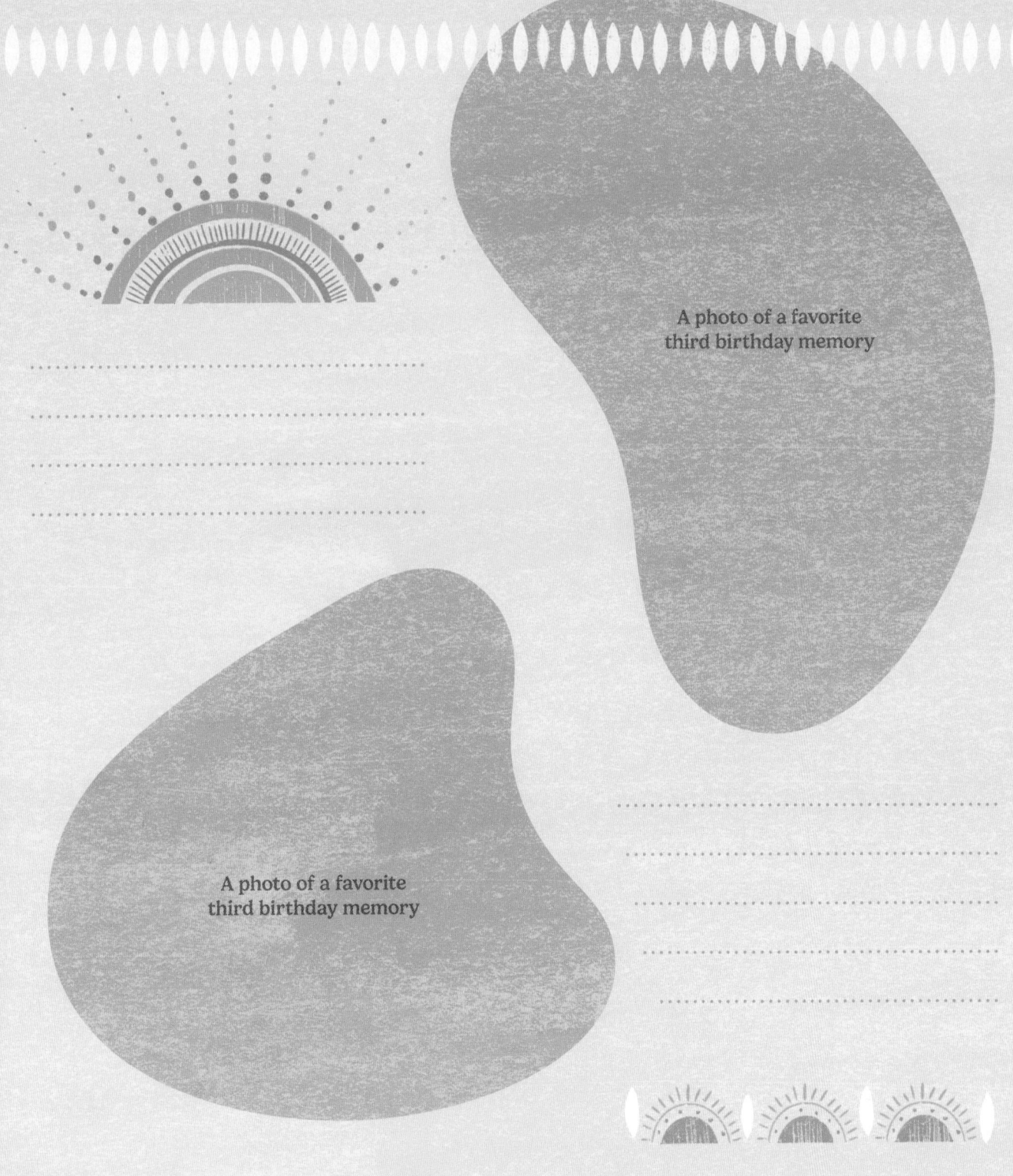

Three Years Strong

These are some highlights from your third year.

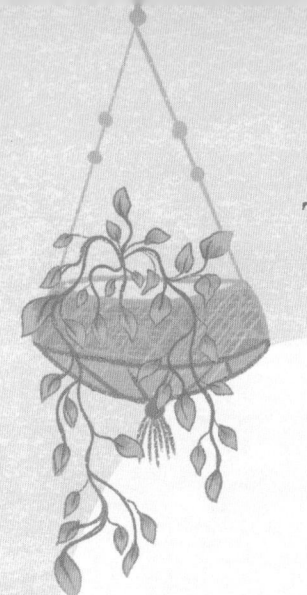

A photo of baby doing something they love

Now you are so good at ....
....
....
....

You are still learning ....
....
....
....

You taught us ....
....
....
....

You love to go to ....
....
....
....

You make others laugh by ....
....
....
....

Your favorite things to do are ....
....
....
....

Some of your favorite people are

....

....

....

A favorite photo from baby's third year

....

....

....

....

Favorite Places

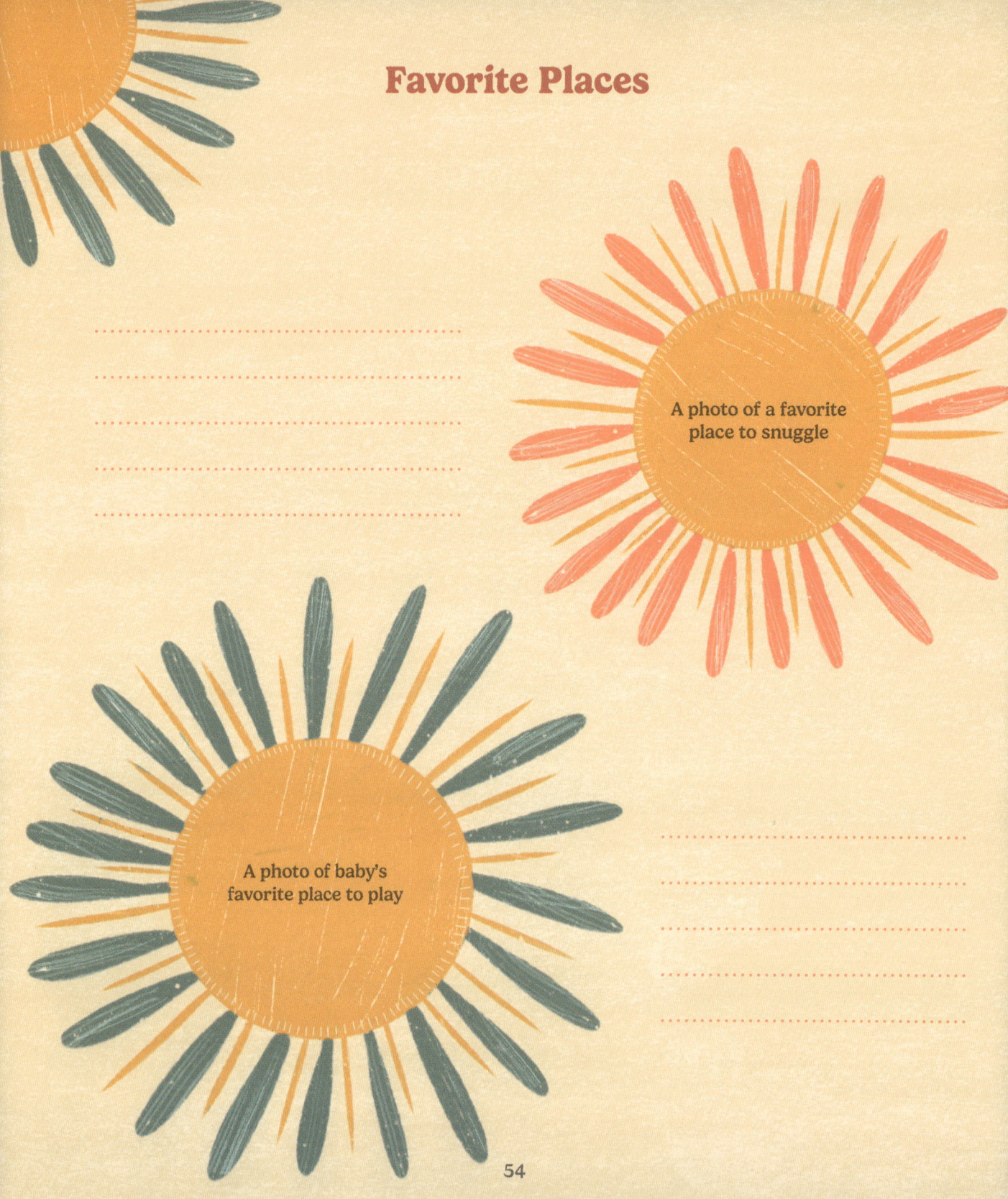

A photo of a favorite family outing

....
....
....
....
....

Beginning with Books

Reading a book that makes baby laugh

Snuggling with a story baby loves to read at bedtime

Reading a book Mom or Dad loved as a kid, too

Baby with all their books

Animal Friends

Baby's favorite animal pal

....
....
....
....
....

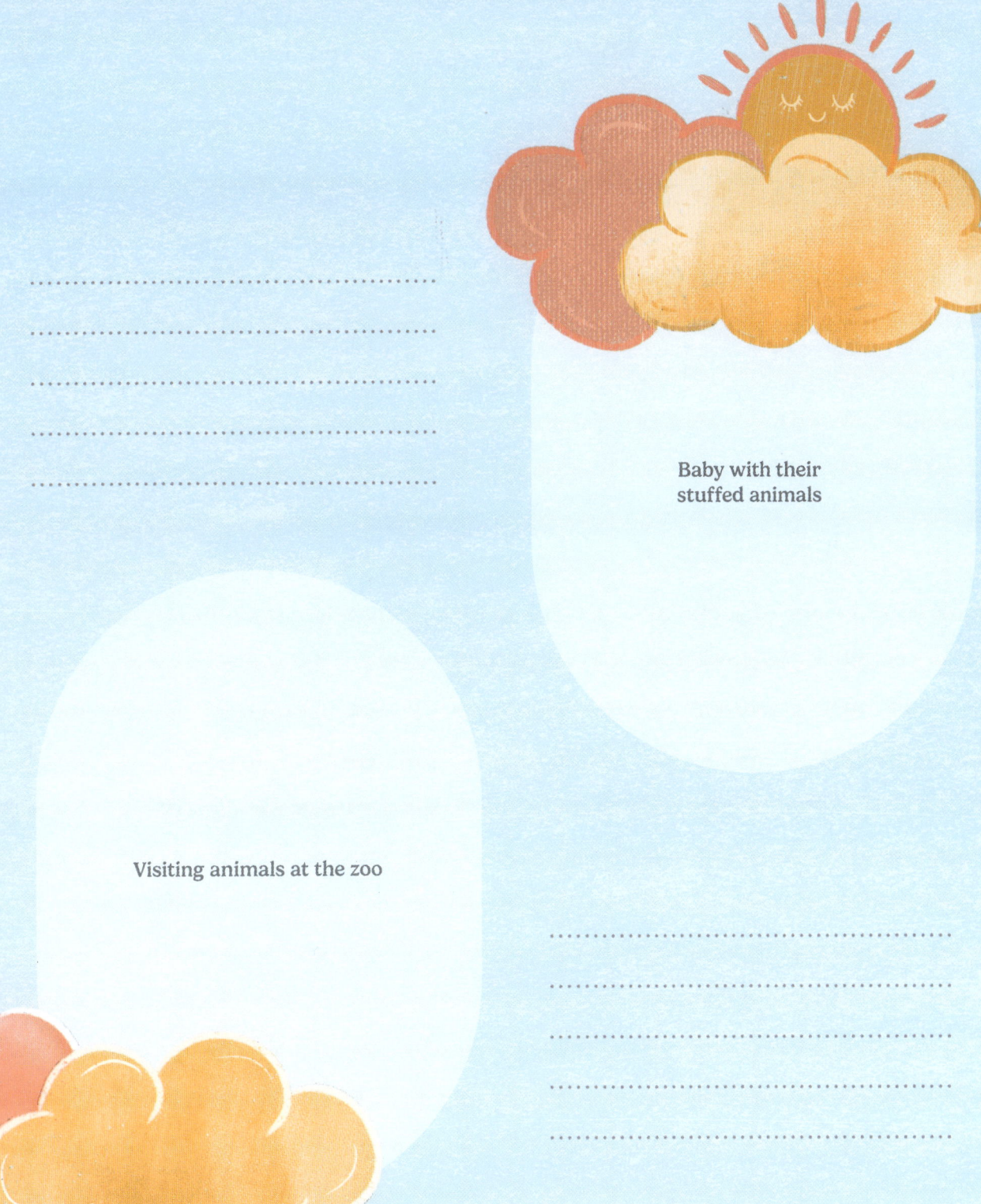

Baby with their stuffed animals

Visiting animals at the zoo

Holiday Moments

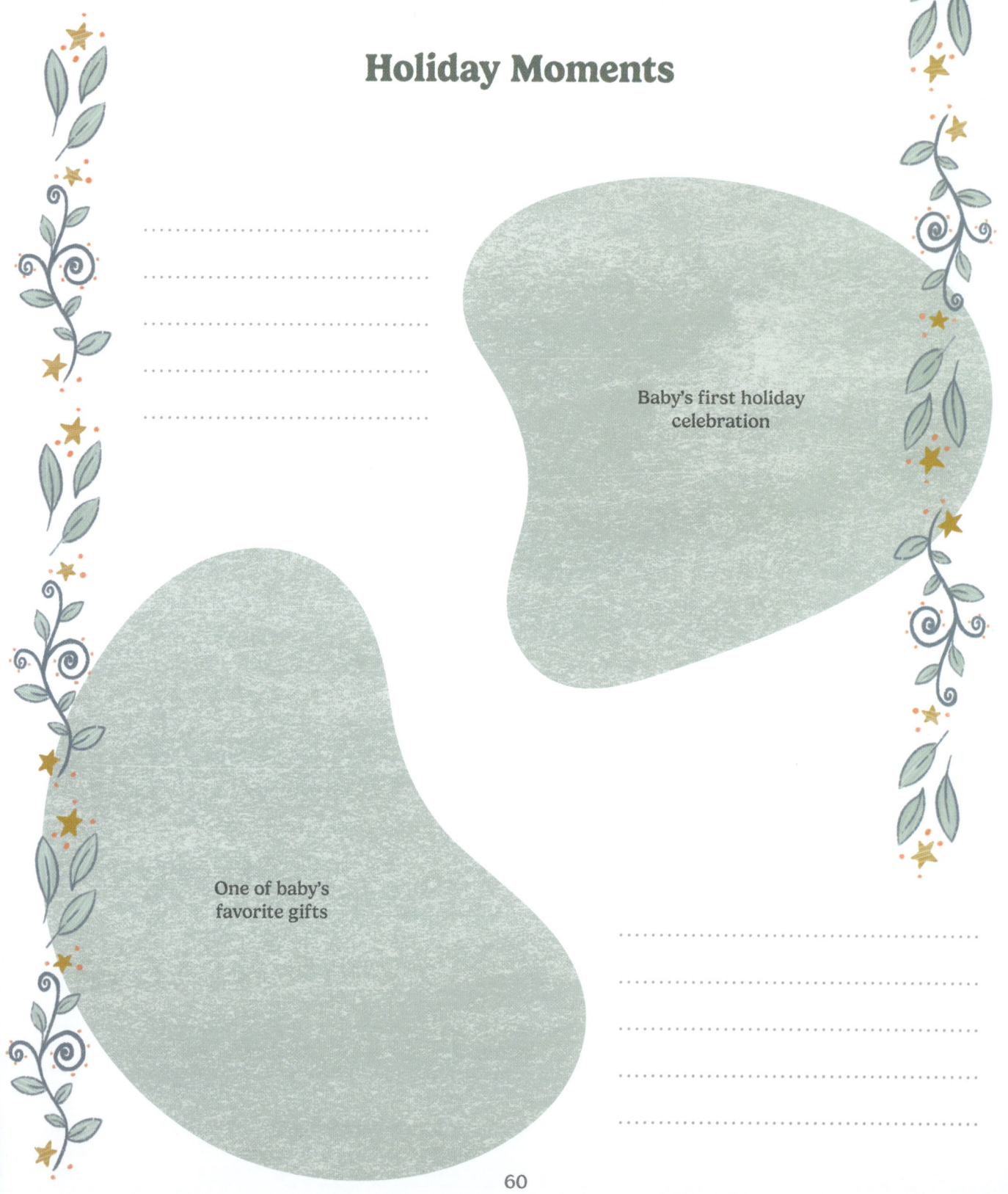

Baby's first holiday celebration

One of baby's favorite gifts

Our favorite way to celebrate together

....

....

....

....

....

A new tradition

A Letter to Future You

A letter to you as you continue growing and loving and exploring and learning...

....
....
....
....
....
....
....
....
....
....
....
....
....
....
....
....
....
....
....
....